D0501831

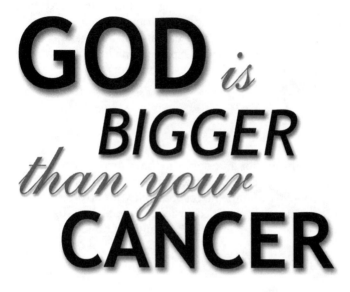

GOD *is* BIGGER *than your* CANCER

**FRESH
WATER
PRESS**

Grover, Missouri

Fresh Water Press
P.O. Box 18
Grover, MO 63040
www.Godisbiggerthan.com

Second printing 2009

ISBN 978-0-9801591-0-3

ATTENTION HOSPITALS, CARE CENTERS, AND PROFESSIONAL ORGANIZATIONS:
Quantity discounts are available on bulk purchases of this book for educational or gift purposes. Special books or book excerpts can also be created to fit specific needs.
For information, please contact:

Fresh Water Press
P.O. Box 18
Grover, MO 63040
www.Godisbiggerthan.com

This book is dedicated
to the
three greatest reflections
of Christ
in my life:

My husband,
  for teaching me about true **sacrifice.**

My son,
  for teaching me about true **joy.**

My daughter,
  for teaching me about true **beauty.**

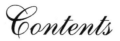

Contents

Chapter One

Why Did God Make Cancer?

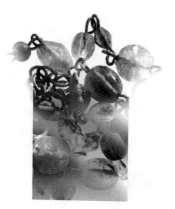

There is no path
ahead *of you*
where He will not go
before *you*

Three Worms and a Slug

When God created the world, why didn't He make it cancer-free? The answer is that He did. When God finished creating the heavens and the earth, He declared that all creation was not just good, but very good, *exceedingly* good. Because Adam and Eve were sinless, they walked with our perfect God in the beauty of the Garden of Eden. No illness, no death, no nausea, no side effects, and no toxins existed there. Yet visible in the background grew the Tree of Good and Evil, and nearby hid the serpent. With the

"To receive

serpent's encouragement, Adam and Eve chose to eat a piece of the forbidden fruit from this tree, leaving all of God's perfect creation tainted by sin. God didn't create cancer. Cancer is a result of living in a fallen, sinful world.

Why did God put that tree in the garden to start with? Why did He give Adam and Eve a choice to obey or disobey Him?

It's kind of like the year my children got me a Christmas present and put it under the tree. In the days leading up to Christmas, they revealed how they had chosen the gift, paid for it, and wrapped it all by themselves. I would have been thrilled if the box contained three worms and a slug; this was the most precious gift I had ever received. On Christmas morning, I opened the box to discover a necklace.

If I had taken them to the store, pointed to the necklace, given them the money, and supervised the wrapping, the outcome would have been the same. I would have received the same necklace. But the true value of the gift was my children's desire to

this priceless gift...

show me their love.

God wants no less from His children. He wants us to turn to Him, but unlike my children's gift to me that Christmas morning, we bring nothing to God, not even three worms and a slug. God provides the gift: grace. Grace is God's gift of salvation for eternity, through Christ's death on the cross. To receive this priceless gift when there is nothing we can do to deserve it is unfathomable. All we do is turn to God and receive this gift. At the same time, in giving us the ability to turn to Him, God also gives us the freedom to turn away from Him.

The down side of this gift is that with this freedom comes a world filled with sin and disease. The up side is that grace makes life worth living. Our ability to turn to God is also our ability to be in an intimate relationship with Him. God could have created robots instead of humans. After all, robots don't get cancer. Robots would have done what they were supposed to do, when they were supposed to do it, and no one would have eaten from that

...when there is

forbidden tree. Robots are great at obedience, but lousy at intimacy.

Because we are free-thinking humans, we have the incredible gift of living on this earth while enjoying an intimate relationship with Jesus. We have the opportunity to continually throw ourselves more deeply into sweet intimacy with our risen Lord. This gift is not left in our fragile hands. Imagine this: our all-powerful God designs all of His plans to draw us deeper and deeper into a relationship with Him. The Lord God Almighty will stop at nothing—*nothing*—to be our intimate Companion, our beloved Savior, and our adoring Father.

Please understand that God hates the suffering that comes with our freedom to receive His grace. From the time sin entered the world, God's single purpose has been to be reunited with His precious children the way He once was with Adam and Eve. In order for us to be with God in His perfect presence, He sent His Son Jesus to pay for our sins. We still have the freedom to receive grace or to turn

nothing you can do...

away. And God still endures the heartbreak when His children reject Him, the anguish of knowing His children suffer, and finally, the agony of sending Jesus to the cross, to gain what He hungers for: the hearts of those He loves.

This message is especially important to you who are suffering from cancer. God has not abandoned *you*, His precious child, in this fallen, cancer-ridden world. Nothing can take Him from your side. There is no path ahead of you where He will not go before you. There is no hospital, no treatment room, and no sick bed where He will not hold you and give you strength. Do not be afraid and do not be discouraged. The Lord God Almighty Himself is with you now and forever.

...to deserve it

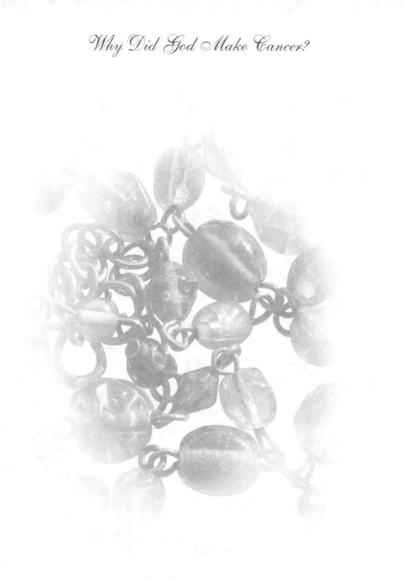

is unfathomable."

The

LORD

Himself

goes before *you*
and
will be with *you;*

He

will ***never*** leave *you*
nor forsake *you.*

Do not be *afraid;*

do not be *discouraged.*

Deuteronomy 31:8

A Meeting With Jesus: Lisa's Story

I knew fear long before I knew cancer. Frightened is no way to live. It almost sounds cliché to say my husband Ken was wonderful, my daughter Rebecca was beautiful, and my home was lovely, but it's true. Yet for weeks at a time I would struggle with the fear of catastrophe if I were alone. I'd become obsessed with "What ifs?" *"What if I have a heart attack in the grocery store?"* *"What if I die at the wheel of my car?"* Eventually I was diagnosed with an anxiety disorder. For the least little thing, I would rush to the emergency room. Driving by myself or leaving the house alone was out of the question, for fear that something terrible would happen. Then something terrible *did* happen: I was diagnosed with Hodgkin's lymphoma.

I kept getting colds that year, but it was a bug bite that wouldn't go away that got me to the doctor's office. When I mentioned the six-week-old cough and the tightness in my chest, my doctor sent me for more tests. He found cancer. For years I had worried that something like this might happen, yet I couldn't believe it when it did. Really, I was in denial. For days I believed it was anything but cancer.

I always felt very close to God as a child, but as an adult battling anxiety, I drifted away from Him. I was not praying, and I began to wonder, *"Are You there, God?"* I was so focused on a future catastrophe that might never happen that I lost sight of God. Despite my weakened faith, God began to lead me over every hurdle from the very beginning of my cancer.

My first hurdle was my doctor's treatment plan for me. As a child, I never wanted to take any kind of medicine for fear it would hurt me. Now they wanted me to have chemotherapy? Just the idea of taking poison to kill part of my body freaked me out. But I was more frightened of the cancer than the treatment. So I began to pray, *"God, give my doctor the wisdom to cure me through You."* So when the doctor said, "Do chemotherapy," I did chemotherapy.

The good part of chemotherapy was that I never had to be alone. For each treatment, Ken sat beside my recliner as I sipped soda and chewed on ice for the nausea. Within a few short weeks, my pain and symptoms from the cancer had decreased. By week six I was already asking, "Are you sure I need to come back for more treatments?" The answer was always an emphatic "Yes!" But they said I *might* not have to undergo radiation.

The thought of radiation renewed my long-time fear of a heart attack. My mother had a history of heart problems, so I worried excessively about my heart long before I was ever diagnosed with cancer. A mild case of heartburn led me to believe I was having a heart attack. That fear would trigger an anxiety attack with such chest pains I thought I would die. Now they wanted to shoot radiation next to my heart with *minimal* risk of heart damage. "The radiation treatment," I was told, "would be the icing on the cake…just what you need to go toward your cure." Again, I was more afraid not to do it than to do it. The worst outcome to me was to skip the radiation and return a year later to discover the cancer was still there, because I had not had the treatment. So I decided to go forward with the radiation.

When I went for my first treatment, they tattooed me with dots so they could make sure they hit the right spot. Then they took me into a sealed room and had me lie underneath a huge machine that looked like a space capsule. It took an hour for eight guys and a nurse to prep me for the procedure. They'd slide me back and forth and mark me up with a Sharpie pen to make sure I was in the right position so the radiation would not damage my heart.

As I lay there, I felt really scared of how much pain the radiation would cause, and then I started to worry about my heart getting damaged. The nurse could tell I was getting more and more scared, so she began to chat to make me feel better. "Do you have any kids?" she asked. The thought of my kids started me crying and I couldn't stop.

My mind kept racing, *"What am I doing here? I could be at school helping out in Rebecca's classroom instead of lying under this machine."* Needless to say, I wasn't holding still anymore, so it was harder for them to prep me. Prayer was the only way I knew to calm down: *"Please, God, protect everything else and just get the bad stuff."* Finally, I settled down enough to go on.

They had me lying down with my hands clasped

together over my head, and they said there would be two intervals of radiation. Then they all walked out, closing this giant bank vault-type door behind them. I was alone. No Ken, no Mom or Dad, not even a nurse or a tech guy. I'm like, *"Oh, my gosh! I'm in here all by myself!"* I'm freaking out and my mind is racing, but I knew if I fell apart again, I'd only be in there longer. So again I prayed, *"Jesus, You're the only One who can be in here with me. You're the only One who can be with me **all** the time. Please, Jesus, hold my hand."* And from my clasped hands, I'd place my right hand out just enough so someone could hold it. I closed my eyes, trying so hard to stay still, and then Jesus was there. I could feel Jesus holding my hand. My body began to relax and my mind calmed down. I felt this wonderful sense of total strength—not just peace, but this empowering strength. Jesus filled my spirit so there was no room for fear. Now I know that you cannot focus on your fear and on God at the same time. I made it through all my radiation treatments, holding my hand out so Jesus could hold onto me.

I'm in remission now, and I wish I could say my

anxiety is miraculously healed, but it's not. The difference now is I've learned ways to cope. When I start to think, *"What if?"* I immediately think, *"No, no, no! I'm going out there and I'm going to have fun! I went through six months of treatments where I missed spending a lot of time with my daughter and doing things other people do daily. I'm not staying home anymore."* It's strange that God could use something as frightening as cancer to teach me how to cope with my fears.

My faith has grown and I feel the same closeness with Jesus I felt as a child. I don't wonder where He is anymore. I know where He is: He's always with me! I know there are frightening places where no one else can go with me…except Jesus. I found a verse that has been my rock to see me through:

> *"The Lord Himself goes before you and will be with you; He will never leave you nor forsake you. Do not be afraid; do not be discouraged."*
> Deuteronomy 31:8

It's true! Jesus will also go with you, and He'll never, *no never,* leave you nor forsake you! So do not be afraid and do not be discouraged. You are not alone.

15

Sweet, precious Lord,

I place myself *fully*
in the **shower**
of Your *abundant* **grace**
and ask for Your **forgiveness**.

I know that I do **not** deserve

to be 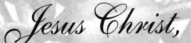 **washed clean**
by the **blood** of **Your Son**,

Jesus Christ,
but as I submit to Your love,

I am.

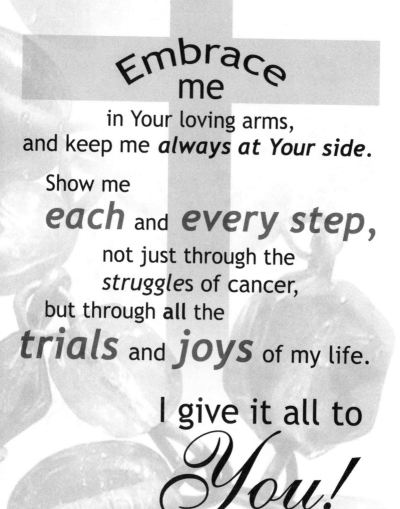

Embrace me
in Your loving arms,
and keep me *always at Your side.*

Show me
each and *every step,*
not just through the
*struggle*s of cancer,
but through **all** the
trials and *joys* of my life.

I give it all to
You!
Amen

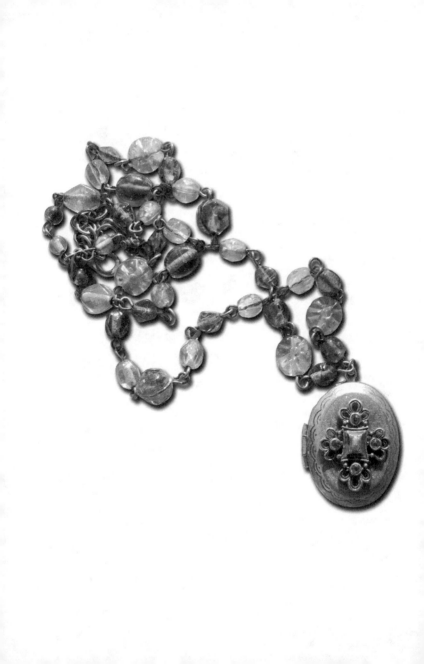

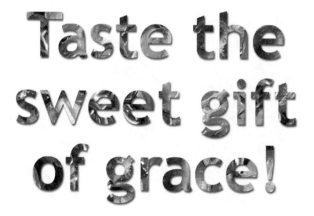

Chapter Two

Is God in Control, Even of My Cancer?

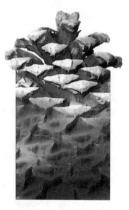

*With God's way,
the **fire**
always ends in
rebirth*

Giant
Pinecone Seeds

You don't know what a nightmare is until you hear the doctor say you have cancer. Before the word *cancer,* your life revolved around work, family, and friends. Now it's governed by treatment plans, white cell counts, and test results. The doctors explain that to heal you they must kill off a part of you. Sure, they're killing cancer cells, but the cells aren't living on a plant in the back yard; they're living inside of you. The worst your body could do to you before was a bad head cold or maybe a nasty stomach flu.

Now you live unsure which side effect will dominate your day.

The nightmare is darker on bad days. The people you used to take care of are now taking care of you. The places you used to go, you can't go, and if you manage to get there, you're too tired to stay. The things you used to do, you can't do, at least not the way you did before. Even on good days there's the chaos of hospital bills, insurance plans, and the cost of prescriptions. How can God be bigger than this nightmare called cancer? If God is in control, shouldn't you be healthy and happy instead of sick and scared?

As strange as it sounds, God does some of His best work when things are dark. Sometimes chaos is part of God's plan. I saw this truth while hiking through the San Bernardino Mountains, outside of Los Angeles. That forest had pinecones as big as porcupines. I grew up in Florida and can remember stepping on those puny pinecones, then pulling out the little seeds. To extract the seeds from California's

"It is through...

giant pinecones requires more than crushing with child-size feet. It requires fire. God's plan for the reproduction of these trees and the continuation of those forests is fire. It is through the destruction of the forest that new seeds are planted and rebirth begins.

This sounds pretty good in textbooks. However, standing in front of a massive forest fire, it is pretty hard to say, *"This is great! Years from now there will be a beautiful forest in place of these ashes."* You question whether any good can come from such devastation. As a human, you don't plan on destruction. You don't plan on losing a loved one, a job, a home, or a marriage. And you surely don't plan on being a cancer patient.

When things don't go according to your plan, it doesn't mean that things are not going according to God's plan. God will use any detour, mistake, or crisis in your life for His purpose. God isn't only in control when things are going fine; God is in control at all times, over all things, in every way. God is in

...the destruction of

control even when you can't see His hand in your life. God is in control even when you doubt if He hears you, knows you, or loves you. Faith is knowing you are still resting in God's mighty right hand, even when it feels like you are free falling into darkness. God is with you. God is holding you. God is in control of all things.

As reassuring as it is to know that God is in charge, even in the chaos, it's also the reason why submitting to God's will is scary. Sometimes His plan requires suffering. God is still in charge; His will is being done, but you or someone you love may have to suffer.

So you resist God's will. If you're like me, you try to implement your own plan to avoid the things you fear. *"If God's not offering any guarantees that no one will suffer, I'll just charge off on my own plan."* The problem is that acting like you're in charge is an illusion. God is even in charge of the people who think they're in charge.

Or maybe your style is to deny the possibility that

the forest that new...

anything can go wrong. *"Everything will be painless because Jesus loves me."* Faith is not that you believe Jesus loves you and won't let you suffer. Faith means you know that if there is suffering, Christ is still in control—even in the midst of your greatest fear.

Imagine your greatest fear coming true. Take a moment to grasp your greatest fear. Picture it with all of its ugliness, darkness, and terror. Is God still there? Is He still in control? Is He still all-knowing and all-powerful? *YES!!*

Hold this promise from God deep within your heart:

> *"For I am convinced that neither death nor life,*
> *neither angels nor demons,*
> *neither the present nor the future,*
> *nor any powers,*
> *neither height nor depth,*
> *nor anything else in all creation,*
> *will be able to separate us from the love of God that*
> *is in Christ Jesus our Lord."*
> Romans 8:38-39

- Is your fear that this disease will leave your body unable to do productive and meaningful work?

...seeds are planted

God uses each one of us as a part of the mighty body of Christ to accomplish great things!! Do not fear.

- Are you afraid that you will die and leave your children with no one to care for them? God loves your children more than you do. It's true. He will never forsake them or leave them. Do not fear.

- Are you frightened that the medical bills will leave you with such a burden that you can't endure? God will be there with you through every struggle. *EVERY STRUGGLE!* Do not fear.

- Are you frightened that although you know the love of Christ, you are not worthy to be with Him for all eternity? Jesus has gone to prepare a place for you. If this were not true, He would not have said it. Jesus is ready for you. Do not fear.

Nothing—not even your cancer—is outside the dominion of God. He has authority over *EVERYTHING.* Through Jesus' resurrection, He conquered all our fears. Praise the Lord God Almighty!

and rebirth begins."

For I am **convinced** that
neither *death*
nor *life,*
neither *angels*
nor *demons,*
neither the *present*
nor the *future,*
nor *any powers,*
neither *height*
nor *depth,*
nor *anything*
else
in *all* creation,

will be able to

separate us

from the

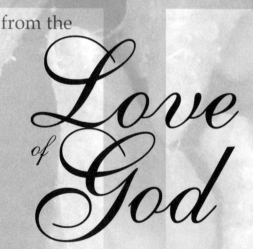

Love
of
God

that is in

Christ Jesus

our **Lord.**

Romans 8:38-39

A Meeting With Jesus: Christina's Story

For reasons known only to Him, God's plan for me was to face the challenge of defeating cancer with an unborn child in my womb, not once, but twice. Jesus came to meet me when I was ready to leave His will for me and take my life, and the life of my child, into my own hands.

At age 35, with three daughters under the age of five, my husband Stephen and I were told I had breast cancer. Suddenly I was overwhelmed with decisions of which treatments to pursue while still striving to do God's will. I decided to pursue non-traditional, natural remedies, because I believed God was going to heal me. After sharing this belief with a friend, she gently said, "Christina, some-times Jesus saves you from the fire, and other times He walks you through the fire." It turned out that God's plan was to take me through the flames.

The flames began small. I had a lumpectomy and the preliminary reports said that they got all the cancer. Four months later, we found out I was pregnant with our fourth child. I was thrilled! I thought all the flames were gone.

Two days later, the doctor told me I had never been cancer-free. There was an unseen final report that said the cancer was still there. I had believed for the last four months that this nightmare was over, when actually the cancer had been spreading through my breast. The flames were still there, only larger.

I was told I couldn't have chemotherapy, radiation, or a mastectomy unless I aborted my son. I was so scared; I even considered my oncologist's strong recommendation to have an abortion. Thankfully, my husband was completely against it. We chose to keep our child and not have any treatments. We knew this was God's plan. So many times I thought I saw God's path for me, only to have the path lead me back into the flames.

Since my cancer was estrogen fed, my pregnancy increased my estrogen, which, of course, increased my cancer. If I received chemotherapy, there was a high possibility that the baby would have leukemia or some form of birth defect. Yet at 16 weeks pregnant, the tumor in my breast had grown to four centimeters. I had no choice but to do something. So I began chemotherapy.

Then I wondered if I heard God wrong when I re-fused chemotherapy or when I decided not to abort my child. Maybe I had not heard from God at all! I had thought that following God's plan would mean no more flames, or at least not this much. When more flames came, I began to question whether I was really on God's path.

At 32 weeks, and after an induction that lasted three days, we were miraculously blessed with a healthy son, Alex. Now the flames were mostly gone, and I was amazed that God had protected my child from all of the toxic chemicals they had put into my body. After undergoing a mastectomy and completing radiation, things finally began to go well. We had a beautiful, healthy son, I was begin-ning to feel like my old self again, and I was cancer-free. My doubt was gone. God's will seemed so clear I could almost touch it.

Ten months after Alex's birth, I was elated to go in for my last reconstructive surgery. Finally I was going to put all of this behind me. But that was not God's plan. In my pre-surgical blood work-up, they discovered I was pregnant. Stephen and I were in total disbelief. From day one I began to worry about the effects of my earlier chemo treatments on this child. At quiet moments, I would find myself asking God to take this child. The risk seemed too high, but I also thought that perhaps the Lord had given us this baby to show me that life will go on. I hoped that God was finally going to give me the pregnancy that I'd always dreamed of: uneventful. But God had not finished taking me through the flames. By the end of this nightmare, He would not only need to lead me, but also to carry me to safety.

At five months pregnant, I woke up one morning with excruciating pain across the top of my back. My cancer had returned, but this time it was in my bones. With that news, I just crumbled inside. I was told that with an abortion and very aggressive chemotherapy, I might get eighteen months to two years to live.

The counsel to abort the baby now grew stronger and harsher. Instead of just my oncologist recommending abortion, I heard the same advice from at least 20 doctors, nurses, and medical professionals. This was just the beginning of temptations being thrown in my face. Even though Stephen knew that he could soon become a single father with four children, he still adamantly opposed an abortion. I was unsure and began to feel desperate.

My oncologist pushed me the hardest for an abortion. He thought I should take my child's life because my life was at risk. "You have four wonderful children. Give yourself a life with them. Christina, if this God that you serve is so merciful and forgiving, He'll forgive you."

I knew he was right that aborting my son was the correct decision physically and medically. I told Stephen what my oncologist said. His only response was, "That crafty serpent." My husband knew that Satan was using twisted religion and medical reasoning to convince me to abort our child.

Although I heard what Stephen said, I was thinking from total fear. I was standing in the flames and I felt God had left me. *"Why has He done this to me? Why couldn't God hear my prayers?"* I was pleading, begging God to take this child so I wouldn't have to. I wanted action, I wanted it now, and I wanted it my way. I was ready to take control.

The next day I was alone, except for Alex, who was sleeping upstairs. I picked up the phone and called an abortion clinic to find out which days they had procedures, how much they cost, and most importantly, if I could use the abortion pill. I was thinking, *"If I could just take that pill, it would be over. People, and especially my husband, would think that I just naturally miscarried."* I hung up the phone and cried and cried.

I had decided I was going to do it. I was going to abort my unborn child. Then Alex woke up upstairs. I held him in my arms and paced back and forth in despair. Then Jesus spoke to me, "The devil wanted this son, just like he wants the one in your womb." I sobbed, knowing it was true. Finally, I reduced my decision down to what does God's Word say? "Thou shall not kill." I could add nothing to the equation to make a godly choice.

When I came back downstairs, I was a different woman. I knew it was Jesus who spoke to me, because He totally changed my heart. For the first five months of that pregnancy, I questioned every day if I had made the right choice to not abort my child. I lived each remaining day of the pregnancy with complete joy that I was pregnant.

After delivering my son Austin prematurely, they

discovered cancer up and down my spine, on my skull, my hips, my arms, and my legs. I even had a spot on my liver and two spots on my lungs. My nightmare with cancer was not over.

I had now delivered my fifth child, and again they told me I had less than two years to live. I was once more completely filled with doubt that I had ever known God's plan for me. My head knew that God was in control, but I was worrying and acting like it all depended on me. Maybe I should have aborted both my sons so my husband would only have three children to worry about. If I had just had a hysterectomy or my husband had a vasectomy. Or if I had not smoked before I was 20. My dark thoughts went on and on. I had godly people telling me I had done something wrong and that God was punishing me. They said I had issues of unforgiveness. I just wanted to know what God wanted me to do, so I could do it and everything would be all right.

Finally, God showed me that's not how it works. God isn't waiting for us to do the right thing so He can make His will happen. God's will is supreme, with or without us. We need to seek His will, but

He doesn't need us to complete His plans.

God can take everything, *even our mistakes,* and use them for His will. You don't have to walk a perfect walk. When you really get it in your heart and in your head that God's in charge, it takes the pressure off of you. Then you know that all the worry in the world isn't going to add a day to your life. I seek God's plan for me through prayer, fellowship, and the Word, and I make the best decisions I can. Then I leave it in God's hands, because thankfully, He's in control, not me.

Today, Alex is four and Austin is two. The doctors said I was supposed to be dead over a year ago. The cancer miraculously left my lungs, and doctors were able to surgically remove the cancer from my liver. I'm not cancer-free, and every couple of months I'm back in the flames, trying to make the best decisions I can. It's easier now because I have given control to God. I know He can use me, even in the midst of my blunders. I continue to be forced through the flames, but I'm not alone and I'm not in charge. Jesus will wrap His loving arms around me and carry me through again.

Lord God Almighty,
When I am
struck
by the *chaos*
around me,

hold me close
in Your **ever-present** arms.

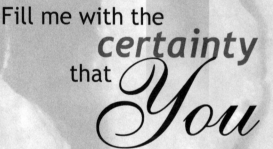

Fill me with the *certainty* that *You* are in **control** of *all things,* at *all times.*

Amen

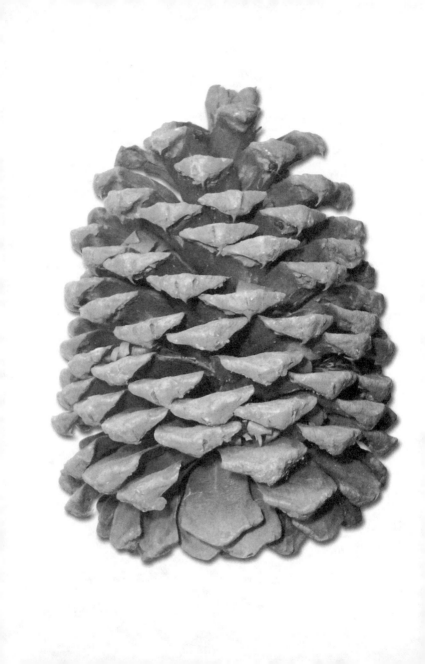

Rebirth begins!

Chapter Three

Why Me?
Why Did I Get Cancer?

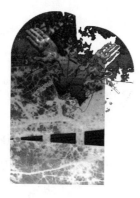

Blessings
from
burdens

The Trials
of a First Grader

*I*t's impossible not to ask, *"Why me? Did I do something to deserve cancer? Is there something I should have done to prevent this?"* As humans, it's easy to dwell on times we did not measure up. *"I should have drunk less soda and more juice." "I should have called my parents more and yelled at my kids less."* Questions about cancer are often directed towards God. *"If only I had gone to church more or prayed more, then maybe God wouldn't have given me cancer." "If only I hadn't done so many things wrong, God would have spared me this* *suffering."* God doesn't work like that. God does not inflict people with cancer.

Maybe your question to God is, *"Why me? I've done so many things right, so how can I have cancer?"* Understand this: living everyday to honor Jesus will not prevent cancer. It would be nice if things were that simple. Since being good can't prevent all struggles, then what does cause the struggles in your life? Perhaps it would help to look at the simple life of a first grader.

As my son Garrett walked from the idyllic time of the childhood paradise known as kindergarten into the adventure of first grade, I heard a door slam shut. No longer were his days filled with playing on the floor and listening to stories as he drifted off to sleep. Now he sat at a desk, completed worksheets, and (dare I say it?) he had homework! The impact was obvious the first day of school, when my unending ball of energy came home from school and lay on the couch until supper. My prodding and the sounds of his friends playing outside could not budge him.

What changed? My son had discovered "work", and he was tired. First grade was hard work.

After a week or two, Garrett's energy level returned. Then he came home with a note from his teacher: *"Garrett was throwing rocks on the playground and will miss recess for one week."* This note was followed by my son's tears, pleadings, and of course, nerve-rattling anticipation of his father coming home. Now my son found more than just work at first grade; he found consequences.

Then came the infamous bus incident. Garrett's school bus stop was the next neighborhood over, so I would drive him to and from the bus stop. One afternoon I was late meeting the bus. Garrett spent the next 45 minutes riding the bus to the end of the line where I met him. As he climbed off the bus tired, frustrated, and scared, there were more tears and pleads, but this time they were mine. Garrett found persecution.

What are the causes for struggles in life? Struggles fall into three categories:

"So rest in the

1. Struggles due to our circumstances.

We live in a fallen world where work, burdens, and cancer are a part of life. Garrett's exhaustion was due to no fault of his own, but rather the fatigue of moving from a half-day kindergarten to a full-day first grade. Cancer is indiscriminate and unfair. Fair would be bad people—like murderers, rapists, and terrorists—getting cancer. Unfair is when cancer hits a mother of young children, a hardworking grandpa ready to enjoy his retirement, an innocent child, a loving sister, or a precious best friend. Cancer is not sent by God, but is a horrendous darkness in this fallen world.

2. Struggles due to disobedience.

We're all tempted and too often choose to do what we desire instead of what God desires. Is there any greater temptation to a six-year-old boy than a rock on a playground? Regardless, this type of struggle is the consequence of our own behavior. Cancer is **not** a struggle of disobedience. Cancer victims do not do anything to deserve cancer.

certainty that...

That's why someone who suffers from it is called a cancer "victim". If you have cancer, God is not punishing you. There is no tally sheet in heaven where God tracks your sins and then punishes you with cancer. Nor is there a list of faithful people that are immune to the darkness of cancer.

3. *Struggles due to conviction.*

We're following the will of God, and suddenly other people's sins cause us pain, even to the point of persecution. My negligence at the bus stop caused Garrett to struggle under no fault of his own. There are some cancer cases which are the result of another person's sin. These are cases where someone has contaminated a work or home environment with no regard to the danger it places on others. Unfortunately, most cancer is not due to a specific location or event; it is a condition of the world in which we live.

Typically, there is no one to accuse and no one to convict for your cancer. This is what leads us to blame God. We want to know *"Why?"*

...*nothing bad*

In Jesus' time, many of God's people believed that having an illness was the result of sin. Jesus' disciples asked Him about a man who was blind since birth, "Who sinned, this man or his parents?" (John 9:2) We could just as easily ask the same of Jesus today.

Imagine Jesus approaching and you asking, "Why, Jesus? What did I do to deserve cancer?"

See Him reach out to you and explain, just as He did to the blind man, "You didn't do anything to deserve cancer. The reason you have cancer is so that the work of God may be displayed in your life." That's right, so God's work can be seen in *your* life. In the midst of your struggles, God will shine through. You may be asking, *"How am I supposed to 'display God's work' for anybody? I'm just hanging on, myself."* Don't worry. It's not your job to figure out how God will shine through you. It's God's job. Your job is to hang on to Jesus the best way you can.

If you hunger to understand how God is using your cancer, it can be frustrating to not see evidence

ever happens...

of God at work. You may only see frustration in the eyes of your family and fear in the eyes of your friends, but no shining ray of God's glory. It's OK if you can't see His glory shining through your life. It's there. God promised. Really! Romans 8:28 states, "…that in all things God works for the good of those who love Him…"

So if God's purpose remains a mystery, rest in the certainty that nothing bad ever happens that God cannot use for good. Just think of it! Even in the midst of a sinful world, God promises to work all things—every stupid, senseless, destructive, and evil thing—for the good of those who love Him. God uses tumors, low cell counts, and even nausea and fatigue to fulfill His purpose. God would not be in complete control if He only used some things or even most things. God *is* in control, and He uses *all* things.

God promises more than showing His works to others. Read Romans 8:28 again. For whom is God working? *YOU!!* God promises to use His authority

…that God cannot

for *your* good! And God knows what is good. He knows we need His goodness; that's why He sent Jesus. Jesus will bring you blessings from burdens and hope from despair. It's true. He will bring *you* blessings from *your* burdens and hope from *your* despair.

Lay your head back and rest in the loving arms of your Heavenly Father. Know that your cancer is not senseless; it has purpose. God's purpose is for His glory to be *revealed* through **YOU**. All praises go to Him. HALLELUJAH!

use for good. "

Do *not* be *anxious*
about **anything,**

but in **every***thing,*
by
prayer **&** *petition,*

with *thanksgiving,*

present your *requests*
to
God.

And the

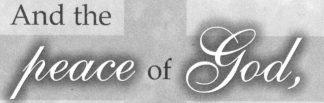

peace of *God,*

which transcends **all**
understanding,

will guide
your
hearts & your
minds

in

Christ Jesus.

Philippians 4:6-7

A Meeting With Jesus: Robin's Story

I 've worked in the nuclear business since 1981—first in construction, then in operations. Last October, when I was diagnosed with prostate cancer, I began to wonder if I'd done something. I've had some radiation exposure, but nothing excessive at all. Unlike others, I've never been one to take those kinds of risks. I feel I haven't been a risk taker, and yet here I was with cancer.

In hindsight, maybe I should have picked up on the symptoms sooner, but they were so subtle that I was lulled into being more passive instead of aggressively discovering the problem. I first had the inkling that something was going on when my urine flow began to slow, and then I had trouble starting to urinate. This lasted over a period of four to five months. One day I'd think, *"It's in my mind,"* or *"I didn't really notice it today."* I began to wonder if the symptoms were real or not real. When I began to see a decrease in semen, I thought, *"I'm 50; maybe I should start expecting this by now. It's not like I'm 21 anymore."*

In October of last year, my loving wife Carla prodded me into getting a physical because I was 50. The exam didn't show anything, but the blood test showed my Prostate Specific Antigen (PSA) test result was high. The doctor said it was probably chronic prostatitis and gave me ten days of an anti-biotic. The second PSA was still high, so he referred me to a urologist.

That's when I found out that my original PSA score was a 38 and the second one was a 31. This was pretty alarming, as the normal PSA results should be less than 4. But the urologist said, "Even with an infection it can be that high. I don't think it's cancer." He gave me 30 days of antibiotics. By then it was around Christmas, so in January I had another PSA blood test performed. It was still high at 28, so they performed a needle biopsy of the prostate.

The results came back to the doctor in a short time. When I went to his office to hear the results, Carla said she wanted to go with me. I told her this was just going to be routine and she didn't need to change her plans just to go. Little did I know that things were not going to be routine for a long time.

When the doctor told me I had cancer, he just said very bluntly, "Hey, there's no good way to say this."

I said, "You don't have to; you just said it." My urologist had taken eight needle biopsies of the prostate.

"The pathology report says that two of the quadrants came back positive," he said. "The cancer is in the upper quadrants and we won't know if it is contained until we perform a bone scan and CT." The pathology report also rated the cancer as fairly aggressive.

I went back for the scans that we had prayed would show the cancer contained in the prostate. The scans would tell us whether the cancer had metastasized in the bones or my lymph nodes. If the cancer was contained, we stood a good chance of getting it with surgery.

From the test results, I had every indication that the cancer had not metastasized somewhere else. My oncologist did a special carbon scan with an affinity for prostate cancer. The results showed cancer in the prostate, but nowhere else. So I elected to do the surgery.

The hard part was not my own dealing with the

cancer. The hard part was seeing the impact on my family. I didn't have any problem when I found out I had cancer. Inside you say, *"Prepare yourself."* The doctor says the word "cancer", then you take a deep breath and say, *"OK, I'm going to deal with this."* The tough part was telling my boys. Eric was a junior in high school. Ryan was still away at college. There's no good way to tell someone you love bad news at a distance.

We called Ryan on the phone once we'd gotten the results back. I had a feeling that he knew from the tone in my voice that the news was not good. I said it pretty much the same way the doctor told me: "There's no good way to say this." Silence hung on the other end of the phone. Then I tried to listen for breathing or anything that could tell me how it was going with him. I could tell that he was having a lot of trouble with this. By the time I hung up, I felt like we had gotten through the worst part of it. Fortunately, Ryan had friends for support at school, and he came home as soon as he could.

Telling my younger son was really hard. Eric didn't take it too well. It took a couple hours before we got things calmed down again. I wasn't ready for that. He comes off as a real tough guy, but he's not. When Eric was young, we'd go fishing, but we never brought any fish home because he wanted me to set them loose. He just couldn't see anything get hurt. Now he's 6-1 and 230 pounds, with a tough outside and a soft middle. He seldom lets people see the middle. I hated seeing what my cancer was doing to my boys.

It's most difficult for me to think about the potential future impact the cancer will have on my family. That's the way I'm wired. I'm more concerned about others. The treatment was nothing. I have a pretty significant pain threshold. The ruptured disk I had in my back a few years ago was much more painful to deal with than this surgery. Having to deal with the realization of what this was doing to my family led me to question, *"Why me? Why now?"*

I had taken care of myself pretty good, I had a good faith walk, and I looked around and said, *"Why do I have cancer? Have I done something?"* I'm a very analytical "process and procedure" type person. I stopped and said, *"I've done all these steps and yet I didn't get the results I expected."*

That's part of the curse of being so scientific and analytic: You feel that with this process or that procedure you have a high probability of a known outcome. But that doesn't always work.

For one thing, I felt like my body had betrayed me. I'd think, *"I've taken care of my body, so what did I do to deserve this betrayal?"* Then I went from denial, *"This is not happening to me,"* to anger, to mad at everything and everybody, to furious about what it was doing to my family. There were times if I wasn't careful, I'd regress and go through these emotional things all over again. I guess it's normal to go through several cycles of these feelings.

I elected to have the surgery; they call it a radical prostatectomy. The pathology report on the removed prostate was not good news. The prostate showed two microscopic focal extensions in the lower quadrant of the prostate. The surgeon said we couldn't be sure that all the cancer was removed during the surgery. He recommended that we perform follow-up PSA testing to monitor my condition.

The first time I went back for a check-up was frightening. The doctor tried to prepare me. "This is early, your numbers were so high; don't expect them to be down." The PSA results came in below detectable. I had surgery on March 15th, and here it was eight weeks later. Wow, the result was below detectable! That's one of those moments you go, *"Whew, I was blessed."* I had goose bumps on my arms and the whole nine yards.

I still keep reliving the *"Why?"* Mentally, I think I have put that behind me and try to move on, but there are still times when it just comes roaring back at me. There are days when I wake up trying to figure out why, and I go, *"Do I have to go over this again? Is this something I have to re-experience?"* I start thinking that in three to four weeks I'll go in for another PSA test, and I pray to God that it comes back below detectable.

Still, from a faith perspective, I don't feel like I'm being punished or that God is doing this to me. I do feel like He is using this and that there is good coming from it. Certainly there's been good for me and for my family, even though it's painful. Of course, I wouldn't say, *"Yes, sign me up! Cancer's a good experience for everybody."*

But it's given me an opportunity to minister in a new way. I was aware of prostate cancer before I was diagnosed, but I did not know what symptoms to look for. I'm more knowledgeable now, and I'm not afraid to share what I've learned. I ask every man that I come in contact with if he knows his PSA number. One out of every six men will have a problem with prostate cancer. We need to be talking about it.

At one of our safety meetings at the facility where I work, I felt moved to testify about my cancer. There were about 80 people there. I tried to educate them about how I found out, and that 45 or 50 is not too young for prostate cancer. We have an aging workforce with a lot of men who are taking their health for granted. I've tried to use my cancer for the positive by reaching other men and making them aware. Heaven forbid that someone else will go through it, but maybe what I have to say will lead to early detection for someone.

What it really comes down to is that "why" doesn't matter. Why me and why now are not important. What's important is to see some kind of good come from this experience. I have seen blessings from it in my life already, and I know there will be more to come.

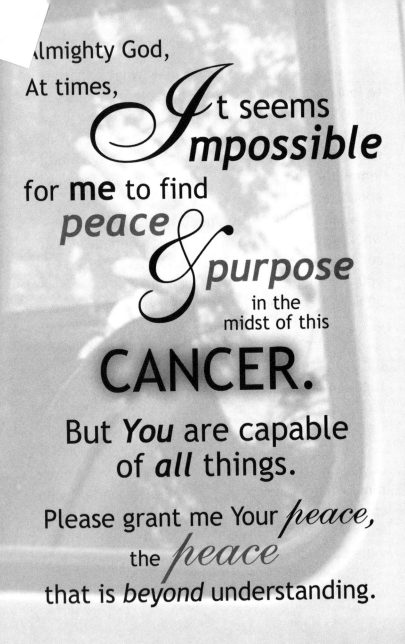

Almighty God,

At times, *It* seems **Impossible** for **me** to find *peace* & *purpose* in the midst of this

CANCER.

But *You* are capable of *all* things.

Please grant me Your *peace*, the *peace* that is *beyond* understanding.

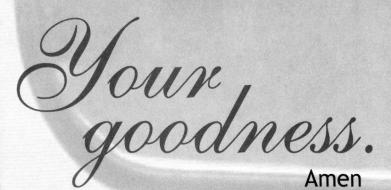

Lift the **BURDENS**

of my

body & **mind**

and let me rest
in the *certainty* of

Your
goodness.

Amen

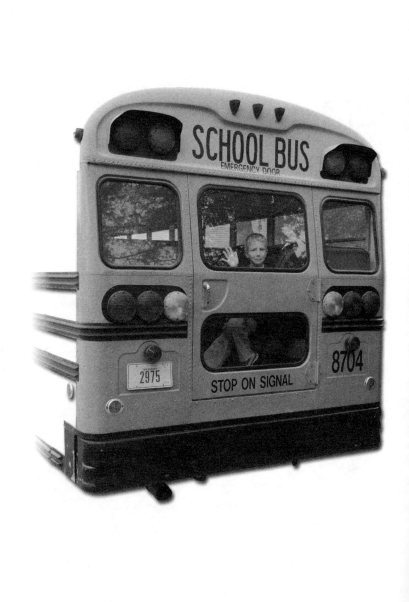

For God's purpose!

Chapter Four

I've Prayed, So Why am I Still Sick?

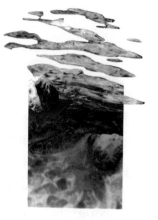

Believe *God knows what is best for you.*
Trust Him.

Bending Water

You believe that Jesus is your Savior and that you will one day be with Him for all eternity in heaven. You believe in the power of prayer and the existence of miracles in our world today. You believe that all things are possible through Jesus Christ our Lord.

You've passionately prayed for a miracle: to have Jesus remove all the cancer from you now and forevermore. But the cancer is still there.

You begin to question; you doubt. Does Jesus heal some and not others?

One evening, after synagogue, Jesus went to Simon Peter's house and healed Peter's mother-in-law. Peter was Jesus' close friend, so you might expect Him to heal the family member of a friend. But then the whole city of Capernaum gathered around Peter's door. And *any* that had diseases were brought to Jesus and He laid His hands on *every one* of them and healed them (Luke 4:38-40). It doesn't say He healed the ones that had faith to move mountains or the ones that prayed the prettiest. Neither did it say that He refused to heal the vilest, most disgusting of sinners. It says He healed them *all*. There is no question that Jesus has the power to heal anyone. Jesus does not refer anyone out to a specialist. He is a one-stop healing machine. Blindness, lameness, leprosy, and demon possession were no problem for Jesus. He even raised the dead. Now, that's a healer!

There's no doubt Jesus can heal your cancer. You probably know a miraculous story of someone who overcame unbelievable odds to survive cancer. So why doesn't He heal everyone like He did that night

"My father taught me...

at Peter's house? Let's look at what Jesus did the next morning.

The book of Luke says that Jesus departed the city and went to a lonely place. The people found Him and tried to keep Him from leaving, but Jesus said, "I must preach the good news of the kingdom of God to the other cities also; for I was sent for this purpose" (Luke 4:42-43). Jesus' mission was not to take care of the people by healing their diseases. His purpose was to spread the good news that God loves them so much He sent His Son to die for their sins. *God's purpose is to be reunited with His lost children.* God gives us miracles so we may believe (John 20:30). But if all Jesus did on earth was perform miracles and not be resurrected, our faith would be hollow. Our faith is not based on Jesus, the miracle worker. Our faith is based on Jesus Christ, the Son of God, dying on the cross for our sins. All answered prayer strengthens our faith, but the source of our faith is the blood of Christ.

We impact God's plans through prayer, but we do

...in a creek

not alter His purpose. When our desires fit with God's purpose, God answers our prayers and fulfills the desires of our hearts. When we are blessed beyond belief, protected without reason, and led to the richness of life, God has fulfilled our desires within the framework of His purpose. If God guaranteed healing, we wouldn't need to pray to God, trust God, have faith in God, or submit to God's will. Submitting to God's purpose or will is asking God for healing, knowing that what we desire may not fit with His purpose.

It's kind of like playing in creeks. Other families have leisure pastimes like biking, camping, or playing softball. Our family plays in creeks. You may be thinking, "Oh, sure. We did that once." Not like us. This isn't a casual activity—this is serious. My kids have grown up playing in creeks, I played in creeks, and even my dad played in creeks. We have a creek-playing season that begins on Mother's Day and ends on that dreaded first day of school. We even have creek shoes. You can't go out and buy creek

a long time ago:

shoes; they have to be the too-small pair of tennis shoes from last summer with your toe poking out of the top to really qualify. We always know when we have a creek neophyte on our hands, because of his store-bought water shoes. We sympathize with his sheltered ways.

So what do you do exactly when you play in creeks? You can hike in creeks, skip rocks in creeks, and even eat lunch on a log in the middle of a creek. But the real creek-playing enthusiast knows the goal is to build a dam, thus creating a small pool in the middle of the creek. After thorough investigation, you select a site with an adequate amount of large rocks in the vicinity. Then everybody takes the biggest rocks they can carry and dumps them in a row across the water. The first rocks dump to the bottom of the creek, and for all apparent reasons, nothing happens. The water continues to rush by as if you'd done nothing. But you keep fetching rocks and piling them on top of each other until you start to see, in one small area, the water begins to slow

You can't

down and create a pool. The excitement in the crew mounts, and more rocks find their way to their rightful place. Finally, the pool expands until the rocks cannot stop the water anymore. The water pushes the rocks down, first in one spot and then another.

That's when I remember what my father taught me in a creek a long time ago: You can't stop the water; you can only bend it. The water has to go downstream. It may go around the dam, through the dam, or even over the dam, but somehow it will get to where it's going.

God's will is like the water, and your prayers are like the rocks, asking the creek to bend one way and then another. When you pray for wisdom, peace, or healing, you're placing a rock in God's will by asking for the desires of your heart. God hungers to fill your every desire, as long as His will still flows toward His reconciliation with His children.

Putting God's purpose above your desires takes your relationship with God to a place where trust, faith, and submission are more than just words. Do

stop the water;

you really believe that God knows what is best for you? Sweet friend, believe these three things:

- God is more than able to heal your cancer.
- God is more than able to protect you through any treatment.
- God is more than able to carry you to your heavenly home in His omnipotent, loving arms.

Trust Him. He hears the prayers you speak, the prayers you think, and especially the prayers you only feel. God will always take care of you, His beloved child.

...you can only

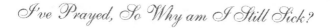

bend it."

This is the
confidence
we have
in approaching
God:

that if we ask
anything
according to
His will,

HE

HEARS US.

1 John 5:14

A Meeting With Jesus:
Irene's Story

I found out last night that the cancer has spread to my other lung. But let's face it, after 22 years of battling cancer, who would have expected I'd hang in there this long? I'm not dead yet! So even if the doctors say, "We have no options," God will work His will. I just figured it's not done until He says it's done. And hopefully that will coincide with me hearing God say, "Well done, good and faithful servant."

In 1985, I was a 39-year-old nurse, diagnosed with stage 1 breast cancer. I woke up one morning and there was a lump in my left breast about the size of my thumb. My doctor said, "This lump is nothing but a fluid-filled cyst."

I don't put my own knowledge above the doctor's, but I do take heed of my own opinion, research, and conclusions. And I know my own body. God was there to tell me to not let loose of my concerns. It was like I had an angel sitting on my shoulder, saying, "Oh...I'm not done with this yet. You keep digging; you keep looking."

With my persistence, my doctor recommended a

surgeon who also said I didn't have a problem and he would check me again in six weeks. Well, at five weeks the lump began to dimple, which is a serious sign of a malignancy. When I went back, the surgeon said, "Removing this lump is a waste of your time and mine."

At that point, I was really digging in my heels and I said, "I want it out!" Finally, he agreed.

Afterward, he came to my bedside and said, "Aren't we glad we got on this right away? It's malignant."

I said, "Yes, we are! Aren't we sharp?"

So that experience taught me that the single best advocate for your health is you. No one is going to help you out and say, "Let me do this dying for you. I'm sorry I screwed up your diagnosis. I'll die; you live." The doctors just don't do that. When there is a mistake made and it comes to the dying that has to be done, you're the one that does it.

It's not always easy being your own advocate. In the nine years between my initial diagnosis in 1985 and my 1994 recurrence, I had other lumps and bumps, and I insisted that each one be removed. The doctors were beginning to get critical of me.

"You can't jump at shadows. You can't live your life obsessed with cancer or in fear of cancer." They were implying that I was educated enough to be more professional. Well, there's nothing professional about having cancer. It's personal.

In 1994, the symptoms of breast cancer began again, but the doctors wouldn't listen. The first symptom appeared in December, when my left breast became much smaller than my right one. My oncologist said it was due to radiation, but then there was some oozing along the scar line in March. My surgeon did a needle biopsy, which has an 11% failure rate. After the biopsy came back benign, I acted really professional and did not cause a ruckus. But over the next months I called my surgeon and my oncologist when my breast began to itch and flake, then ooze and bleed. Then the nipple began to be tucked under and bleed all the time.

In December at my regular appointment, the doctor said, "That's malignant and has to come out right now."

I said, "I've been telling you that for a year."

They diagnosed me with stage 3B inflammatory

breast cancer, which has a five-year survival rate. That was difficult to hear because there are only four stages. With 3B you're standing with one foot on the cliff and the other on a banana peel, and I didn't like being there. So I immediately got five second opinions. I told the five doctors that I was there to interview them for a job. I figured if they couldn't handle that kind of an approach, then maybe I didn't need to be with them anyway. Now, that's not to say that's right for everybody. Some people would go screaming for the hills and say, "I could never do that!" But that's the way I needed to do it. They did a mastectomy on that right side and chemo was mandatory.

Six years later, in 2000, I found a small lesion on my chest that looked like an age spot. For this one, the angel just didn't crawl on my shoulder; she screamed in my ear, "You're not done with this yet!"

My surgeon said, "It won't be anything, but I'll remove it in two weeks."

I said, "I had something a little sooner in mind—like this afternoon. I'll climb up on the table and bring the butcher knife if you don't have one."

When the doctor called with the results, she said, "Irene, I can't imagine what made you insist on having it removed; there's cancer under it." So that immediately put me at stage 4. I went through a very rigorous course of radiation to beat the cancer in 2002. Yet in 2004, a CT scan discovered lesions in my liver.

Liver cancer was really frightening because you can't live without a liver, and there's only so much you can do without damaging it. My two liver surgeries to remove the right lobe in 2004 and 2005 didn't stop the spread. So my doctor pulled a rabbit out of the hat, and I had a special radiation procedure that killed the tumors in my liver. However, when I did the follow-up scans, they found cancer in my left lung. The last two years I've spent searching for something that will work, but to no avail. After trying the latest drugs on the market, I went on a clinical trial, but was unable to stay on. My bone marrow was too exhausted from all the chemo and radiation treatments over the years. They did scans last Monday and found out that it's in both my lungs and in scattered small nodules throughout my lungs. I'm on a hormone treatment now, but we're exhausting my options, because I've become chemo resistant. I get the toxic effects, but not the beneficial effects of chemotherapy. We're hoping the hormone therapy will be effective, but beyond that, there isn't much out there for treatments. However, if it's out there to be found, I'm confident my doctor will find it. He has been a miracle-worker to this point, but, realistically, there is only so much medical science can do.

So that's where we are right now. Twenty-two years of dealing with this, and I feel very blessed to be here. When I was diagnosed at 39, I never thought I'd be here this long. Then some days I think, *"How did I get here so fast?"*

With cancer, some people turn toward God and some turn away. For me, the worse things got, the more I understood that the struggles were a request from God to trust Him, to lean on Him. It was as though God said, "Surrender your trust to Me. I have a plan."

It's funny. On the one hand, God has taught me to fight for the care and treatment I need. On the other, He has taught me to submit. Submit, submit, submit. It's like, *"Well, God, why did You give me free will if You wanted me to submit?"* But it's a different kind of submission. It's not something you give up; it's something you acquire.

A couple of Lenten seasons ago, I decided I'd surrender my will to God. Not just for Lent, but for all time. Usually I would give up something like chocolate. I told Jesus, *"Surrendering to You is probably not going to work out for either of us, because I'm such a micromanager. But this is a once-and-for-all gift."*

It's hard to explain how wonderful surrender really is until you've experienced it. I don't worry about outcomes and decisions. I pray for what I'd like to see happen, but I always say, *"Your will be done and not mine."* It's a daily discipline because I do have a tendency to have a hand in everything. If you can just keep from reaching out and grabbing on to that desire to be in control, and if you open your hands to Jesus instead of closing them, there'll be a huge release of tension. It'll create a lot of space in your life to appreciate the things around you instead of being caught up in the details.

I will tell you that with this last diagnosis, there were some tears and some sadness. Still, God has put me in a place of spiritual trust. I think I know which way His plan is going and I'm not too happy about that. Believe me, I've expressed my anger to God about it. But He has put me in such a place of peace that I don't think about my prognosis too much. I think about what I'm going to do that day. Am I going to work on one of my projects, or go see my friends from church, or maybe visit the grand-kids? It all revolves around living in the moment. It took me years, and I mean years and years, just to learn to get into the moment.

No one gets out of here alive. We're all going to walk this same path. That's not to say I don't fully believe in miracles and that they still happen all around us. I've volunteered numerous times to Jesus to be on the miracle list, but I don't think that's what He has in mind for me. I think I'm sup-posed to be an example, a witness, that if we do love God and truly accept His plan for us, there will be times when that plan does not agree with our plan. That's when we return the love that He's shown us.

I think there are a lot of different ways to ap-proach dying. Some people get depressed. And there is that inescapable sadness of separating from those we love. But what could be so bad about an eternity of praising Jesus? So maybe He can use my life as an example to others of a way to live in joy, with His love, trusting Him and His plans, even if it's not the answer to the prayer that I want.

Maybe...

...my life will
  even make it easier for
    someone else.

All-powerful God,

If it is Your will, Lord,
heal me
of this cancer.

Remove any trace
that cancer
ever resided in my body
as a testimony
to Your mercy
and graciousness.

But if healing
is not Your will for me...

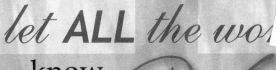

*let **ALL** the wo*

know
that

You

have **NOT**
abandoned
me.

For You are carrying me
through the fire
to be with You always
in heaven
and **on earth.** Amen

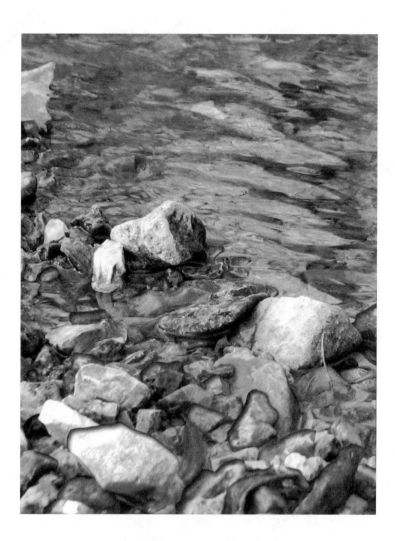

Let God's will flow through you!

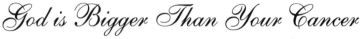

God is Bigger Than Your Cancer
BIBLE STUDY

The mission of this book is to try to answer cancer patients' questions of God. Your questions at times of crisis are opportunities for you to throw yourself at Jesus' feet and let Him lead you through your doubts. Don't let your doubts frighten you. On the other side of your doubts lies a stronger faith. I pray this book helps you to acknowledge your doubts, fears, and anger, and more importantly, to be empowered through Christ's desire to lead you closer to Him. The truth is…God is bigger than your doubts.

It is presumptuous of me to try to answer questions meant for God. After burying myself in God's Word, my hope is to answer these questions by trying to look at cancer and illness through God's eyes. How does cancer fit into this world, God's purpose, and your life?

To further explore these ideas, I have written three

stories, taken from Scripture. Each story is of a man seeking Jesus for healing—sometimes for himself, sometimes for someone else. These stories attempt to show how to view any illness from the perspective of the cross. How was the illness in each story used for God's purpose to be reunited with His children?

Scripture does not tell what happened to these people after the resurrection. Based on what is known about the early church, I have added some plausible solutions to this question.

- The blind man is in Jerusalem for the resurrection.
- The doubting man is present for the miracle of Pentecost.
- As for Lazarus, Scripture does not say what he experienced in heaven. I have used Isaiah's account of being in the throne room of God as my reference.

At the end of each story are several questions for you to explore alone or in a group. My prayer is that this process will continue to draw you closer to your Lord. Amen

The Blind Man

John 9:1-38

*Y*ou wonder if we have met before? Possibly. You see, for most of my life I met people I had never seen. I was the blind man who sat over there, just inside that gate to the city. Yes, now you recognize me. Have you heard that Jesus of Nazareth healed me? Who else could do such a mighty work of God? So surely you heard what the Pharisees did when they heard that a man, blind since birth, was healed? No? Are you also walking to Galilee? Good, then let's walk together and I'll tell how the blessing I had been praying for my whole life was used by treacherous men for evil.

Before I met Jesus, I had certainly heard of Him. People forgot that just because I could not see did not mean I could not hear. Some thought Him simply a rabbi; others firmly believed He was the long-awaited Messiah, the King of Kings. All of Jerusalem was in an uproar when Jesus threw the money changers out of the temple, not to mention when He fed five thousand people from practically nothing. I cared little about these events and whether Jesus had come to raise an army to reclaim Israel. I hungered only to hear of His healings. Leprosy, demon possession, and even blindness disappeared at this man's words. Such a miracle worker! As my lips begged strangers for their scraps, my heart begged God to send this Jesus to heal my eyes.

Then one Sabbath morning, my prayers were answered. As I sat by the gate begging, I heard a crowd approaching. A man's voice asked, "Rabbi, who sinned, this man or his parents that he was born blind?" The crowd stopped and I knew they were speaking of me.

Someone spoke up, saying, "Yes, Jesus, tell us." My mind exploded! Jesus? Could this be the Jesus I had been searching for?

Then a gentle voice reached my ears, "Neither this man nor his parents sinned, but this happened so that the work of God might be displayed in his life." I was stunned by what He said. All my life I had been a pitied figure, not simply because I am blind, but because my blindness was evidence of some terrible sin, either of my parents or myself. No one in his wildest dreams would think that this suffering I have endured was for God's glory. I was speechless.

"As long as it is day, we must do the work of Him who sent me," Jesus said. "Night is coming, when no one can work. While I am in the world, I am the light of the world." He had come to do His Father's work, but could that mean me? Could Jesus be walking down my street on this hot Sabbath morning to meet *me*?

He knelt down beside me and spit on the ground, made some mud and put it on my eyes. "Go," He told me, "wash in the Pool of Siloam." Frightened but excited, I ran to the pool and washed away the mud, and it happened. First, delicate rays of light shattered the darkness. I threw my hands over my face and screamed, unable to grasp what was happening. When I looked again, I saw smoky shapes and then movement; I could see things moving! After several moments, I could tell the shapes were people staring at me and pointing. All I could think of was finding Jesus and throwing myself before Him. But I had never seen Him; for that matter, I had never seen anyone before. I began to stumble back through the streets of Jerusalem. Streets I had walked my whole life in darkness now suddenly came to life in light. From the vendors' stalls came voices I had known so well, but now I could also see the vendors with my own eyes. Tears rolled down my face.

As I drew nearer my street, I noticed a woman pointing at me. "Isn't this the same man who used to sit and beg?" I recognized her voice as the woman who sold olives nearby.

The group around her agreed that indeed I was. But others said, "No, he only looks like him."

I insisted, "I am the man."

"How, then, were your eyes opened?" they demanded.

By now I was beginning to draw a crowd.

I replied, "The man they call Jesus made some mud and put it on my eyes. He told me to go to Siloam and wash. So I went and washed, and then I could see." Once I spoke the name of Jesus, the crowd seemed to change. My healing no longer amazed them. Trepidation seemed to set into their eyes. Weeks before I had heard that the Jews in power had decided that if anyone acknowledged that Jesus was the Christ, he would be put out of the synagogue. It would be nearly impossible to live in Jerusalem and be excommunicated from other Jews. From whom would you buy food? With whom would you do business? How would you live, never setting foot in God's temple? Since the ruling, everyone in Jerusalem was still talking about Jesus, only they were doing it in whispers.

"Where is this man?" one asked me.

"I don't know," I said.

I never knew before that moment that a man's face could speak more than words. His face shouted his fear. With a firm hand he touched my arm and said he was taking me to see the Pharisees. The Pharisees are a powerful group in our Jewish governmental body—the Sanhedrin. I was confused by the man's reaction, but then I realized it was the Sabbath. Jesus had broken a Jewish law by healing on the Sabbath. In the eyes of this man, my healing and my blessing were evidence of Jesus' crime. Several in the crowd joined him and we went to see the Pharisees.

There I stood, in my beggar's clothes, with the stains

from my tears of joy still on my face, being interrogated before these powerful men. I told them how I was healed. Then a debate concerning Jesus began. Some of the Pharisees said, "This man is not from God, for He does not keep the Sabbath."

But others asked, "How can a sinner do such miraculous signs?" So they were divided.

Finally, they turned back to me. "What have you to say about Him? It was your eyes he opened."

I replied, "He is a prophet." This was not the answer they wanted. They wanted some evidence or testimony that would prove Jesus was an ungodly man.

Then they questioned whether I had really been blind, so they sent for my parents. "Is this your son?" they asked. "Is this the one you say was born blind? How is it that now he can see?" This was the first time I had ever laid eyes on my parents and it pained me to see them so frightened.

"We know he is our son," my parents answered, "and we know he was born blind. But how he can see now, or who opened his eyes, we don't know. Ask him. He is of age; he will speak for himself."

The Pharisees summoned me a second time. "Give glory to God," they said. "We know Jesus is a sinner."

"Whether He is a sinner or not, I don't know," I replied. "One thing I do know: I was blind, but now I see!" They really didn't like that response.

Then they asked me, "What did He do to you? How

did He open your eyes?"

Angered that they were trying to set a trap for Jesus, I answered, "I have told you already and you didn't listen. Why do you want to hear it again? Do you want to become his disciples too?"

Then they hurled insults at me. "You are this fellow's disciple! We are disciples of Moses! We know that God spoke to Moses, but as for this fellow, we don't even know where He comes from."

I was outraged that these men were trying to use this magnificent blessing I had received from God for their own evil purpose. I lashed back at them, "Now, that is remarkable! You don't know where He comes from, yet He opened my eyes. We know that God does not listen to sinners. He listens to the godly man who does His will. Nobody has ever heard of opening the eyes of a man born blind. If this man were not from God, He could do nothing."

The Pharisees replied, "You were steeped in sin at birth; how dare you lecture us!" And they threw me out.

I wandered the streets, not knowing where to go or what to do. I felt rejected by man, yet I felt blessed by God. What good had come from my being healed? Every new wonder my eyes drank in was tainted by the thought that this priceless gift was being used to try and destroy the godly man who healed me.

Ahead in the crowd I saw a man looking for something or someone. Our eyes locked and He smiled. Placing a tender hand on my arm, He asked, "Do you believe in the Son of Man?" That voice was the same voice of the man who healed me: Jesus of Nazareth.

I grabbed His arm and asked, "Who is He, sir? Tell me, so that I may believe in Him."

Still smiling, Jesus said, "You have now seen Him; in fact, He is the one speaking with you." My breath caught in my throat as tears drained from my eyes.

When speech returned, I muttered, "Lord, I believe." My knees gave way and I fell at His feet. He lifted me up and took me with Him. I spent that day and many more with Jesus, being filled by His words and His presence. Yet not a day went by that I did not think of those evil men plotting against my Lord. I could not think back on that glorious day when Jesus gave me sight without a feeling of guilt. My good fortune was used as evidence in their plot against Jesus. I never understood why God let that happen—until last week.

You see, the Pharisees' plot worked. They eventually tried Jesus, found Him guilty, and had Him crucified. I could barely believe the horror of His death. All of us who loved Jesus knew that Israel was doomed. Jesus was our last hope. But we were wrong, so wrong. God had a plan. The evil ways of men had been used to show the glory of Jesus. My blindness and my testimony were not horrible mistakes. They were used by God to take Jesus to where He had to go. God knew there had to be a devious plot, a guilty verdict, and finally the cross. Without the cross, Jesus would not have been placed in a tomb and resurrected again in three days.

Jesus' death on the cross was not the end, but the beginning. It was the beginning of a life of knowing that Jesus has conquered sin and death and is now preparing a place in heaven for us. How amazing is that? My blindness, my healing and my testimony were not about me. It was never about me. It was all about Jesus, and God's plan to save His people. Praise the Lord God Almighty!

1. *How do you think the blind man felt as he stood before the Pharisees, being questioned because he was healed?*

2. *Think of a time you knew Jesus was there for you. Maybe it's a blessing in your life or a difficulty He helped you overcome. How would you respond if you had to defend Jesus in a court of law for being there for you?*

3. *How you view your cancer can change from day to day or minute to minute. Some days the fear of cancer fills your entire vision. Other days, the blessings in your life outshine your fears. God sees both, all the time. How do you think God makes sense of your fears and your blessings?*

4. *"For My thoughts are not your thoughts, neither are your ways My ways," declares the Lord. "As the heavens are higher than the earth, so are My ways higher than your ways and My thoughts than your thoughts." (Isaiah 55:8-9)*
   What do these verses mean to you?

The Doubting Man

Matthew 17:14-20; Mark 9:14-29;
Luke 9:37-43; Acts 2:1-41

*H*ey, you there! Have you heard the news? Look around. Three thousand grown men are walking the streets of Jerusalem. Tears of joy streak down our faces. God certainly has an outrageous way of doing things. Of course, it takes something outrageous to get the attention of someone like me.

I have never seen a day of miracles like this! No, that's not true. There was the day Jesus healed my son. Do you want to see a miracle? Then come with me and I will take you to my son. He should not be alive, much less be a strong, healthy, young man. I owe it all to Jesus. Come, you must meet my son, and along the way I will tell you how this whole miracle thing began.

I had little use for miracles until my son began to have seizures. I had always been a self-sufficient man, with a wife, a home, a business, and all the responsibilities those entailed. Fortunately, through my hard work and intelligence, I was successful. Rarely did I run into a situation

I could not tackle. But seizures? What could I do to stop seizures? My own helplessness was the most difficult thing about having a sick child. To watch my precious son suddenly throw himself on the ground, foam at the mouth, grind his teeth, and then become instantly rigid humbled me beyond compare.

Emotions aside, I approached the problem of these seizures like any other: find an expert and have the problem fixed. There is not a doctor in all of Caesarea Philippi that I did not consult. Some pretended to know how to help with an ointment or a potion, but they were useless. With time, the episodes became worse. There was nothing to keep him from throwing his body into a fire or sinking to the bottom of the lake. Really, you will see the scars from the flames when you meet him. I turned to the elders at the synagogue. They said the seizures were from an evil spirit in my son and suggested I call out to God for mercy. I'm a temple-going man, but I wouldn't say I'm a religious man. Spirits and praying seemed unrealistic. I needed a concrete solution.

Could a rabbi from Galilee be the solution we need? I doubted it. Why should He be any different? Word of this Jesus of Nazareth had reached the northern region where I live. Tall tales of the blind seeing and the lame walking raised my hopes. I ached to free my son from his despair. When word came that Jesus and His followers were a half-day's travel away, my son and I set off.

After I found His group on the outskirts of a town, I

wasted no time pleading, "Please take me to Jesus of Nazareth." He was gone. No one could say where He was or when He'd return, but all agreed He would return soon. Then my son began to gag, and down went his body to the ground as the crowd stared in shock. I yelled, "See! This is why I have come! Can no one help my son?"

Several of Jesus' disciples stepped through the crowd and said they would help. Many in the crowd fell to their knees and prayed, as a disciple began to entreat God to free my son from this evil spirit. The more he spoke to God, the worse my son convulsed. It was as though my son was repulsed by anything godly. I finally understood that something evil had grabbed hold of my son. The frightened reaction of the crowd told me that my son was more than any of them bargained for. I crumbled to the ground in frustration, thinking this was useless, just another dead end.

Then a scribe began to taunt the disciple, insisting he had no power over evil spirits. My son was not a topic for debate, but a tortured soul lying withered on the ground. That fact did not stop a heated discussion erupting in the crowd, until someone yelled, "It's the Master! He has returned!" The elation from the crowd at Jesus' return was contagious. I began to think there was still hope, and maybe He could help my son in some small way.

I found myself begging for my son at Jesus' feet. "Teacher, I beg you to look at my son, for he is my only child. A spirit seizes him and he suddenly screams; it throws him into convulsions so that he foams at the mouth. It scarcely ever leaves him and is destroying him. I begged your disciples to drive it out, but they could not."

Jesus took in the whole scene: the scribe, the disciples, and my son. "O unbelieving and perverse generation," Jesus said, "how long shall I stay with you and put up with you?" He spoke with such power and authority; I began to wonder if maybe this Jesus *could* heal my son. He turned to me, "Bring your son here."

Several men helped me take my son to Jesus, but when the spirit saw Jesus, it immediately threw the boy into a convulsion. He fell to the ground and rolled around, foaming at the mouth.

Jesus' eyes melted at the sight of my son's agony. He asked me, "How long has he been like this?"

"From childhood," I answered. "It has often thrown him into fire or water to kill him. But *if* You can do anything, take pity on us and help us." Jesus turned His eyes from my son and onto me.

"*If* You can?" said Jesus. "Everything is possible for him who believes." It was not until He said it that I heard it. "*If*"! I had said, "*If*"! I panicked that my offense meant Jesus would disregard my son.

Immediately I exclaimed, "I *do* believe; help me overcome my unbelief!" I wanted to believe that this man could save my son from a life of agony. I held my breath, not knowing what Jesus would do.

Jesus rose and addressed my son, "You deaf and mute

spirit," He said, "I command you: come out of him and never enter him again."

The spirit shrieked, convulsed my son violently, and came out. My son looked like a corpse, and many said, "He's dead." But Jesus took my son by the hand and lifted him to his feet. At first my son was dazed and disoriented, but then he recognized me and smiled—not a face-changing smile, just a gentle smile. I pulled my son to me and wept. We were surrounded by shouts of praises to God and cries that Jesus was truly the Chosen One, the Messiah. I could barely take it all in; I saw only the clarity in my son's eyes. Surely this miracle must have come from God.

My son and I stayed with Jesus and His followers until they moved south again. I heard many things about the ways of God and the ways of man. I believed that Jesus was a man sent by God with the powers to heal anything. But the Messiah? The Christ? I just didn't know. The more I heard Jesus speak, saw His manner, and witnessed the devotion of His followers, the more my doubts diminished. I began to live in the land of "maybe". Maybe He is the Messiah. Maybe He has come to save Israel from the tyranny of Rome. Maybe He is the Way to God the Father. I did not know what to believe, but I did find a hole in my spirit that all my logic and problem-solving could not make go away. Even after He left, Jesus never seemed to be far from my thoughts.

As required by Jewish law, my son and I traveled to

Jerusalem for all the festivals. I'll never forget last Passover when I heard the news that they had crucified Jesus. Some said they were trumped-up charges, while others thought Jesus was a traitor to Israel, trying to start a rebellion. The confusion of trying to make sense of the man I met with the stories I heard was overwhelming. I couldn't believe the terrible things they were saying, but I didn't know what to believe.

The next thing I knew it was Pentecost. So here I am in Jerusalem for the festival, along with Jews from every nation under heaven. This morning, my son was busy so I decided to visit an old friend. As I passed through this neighborhood, a deafening sound like a blowing, violent wind fell from above. It seemed to land on a house on this very street! It shook me to my feet and I almost lost my step. Once the noise lessened, I heard voices from inside the house, shouting and praising God. The voices were not in Hebrew, but in Egyptian, the language my mother had taught me as a child. I saw that the men in the house were followers of Jesus of Nazareth, whom I had met in Caesarea Philippi. Utterly amazed, I asked a man next to me, "Are not all these men who are speaking Galileans?"

He looked from the men to me, and back again. "Yes, I know for a fact they are."

"Then how is it that each of us hears them speaking in his own native language?" I asked.

Looking around, I saw men who were Parthians,

Medes, and Elamites. Some were even from Mesopotamia, Judea, and Cappadocia. There were visitors from Rome—Jews and converts to Judaism—declaring the wonders of God in their own tongues! Amazed and perplexed, the entire crowd was asking one another, "What does this mean?"

Some made fun of them and said, "They have had too much wine."

Then Peter, this big, burly fisherman I had met before, stood up with Jesus' eleven disciples, raised his voice, and addressed the crowd: "Fellow Jews and all of you who live in Jerusalem, let me explain this to you; listen carefully to what I say. These men are not drunk, as you suppose. It is only nine o'clock in the morning!"

Peter went on to explain that Jesus was more than a rabbi and a miracle worker. He was the Chosen One! The Christ! And we Jews, in our ignorance, crucified Him like a common criminal! He spoke of Scriptures that proved it all to be true! When I realized that I had walked and eaten with the Chosen One of God but believed Him not, my shame seeped out of my every pore. There could be no mercy for an unbeliever like me. I was doomed to be shunned by God the Father forever.

But then Peter went on. Jesus was not dead and decaying in a tomb. He had risen from the dead, as King David had said centuries ago. The prophecies are being fulfilled before my very eyes! What did the man's un-explainable speech mean? The Holy Spirit was being poured out by Jesus to His followers. Finally, Peter said, "Therefore let all Israel be assured of this: God has made this Jesus, Whom you crucifed, both Lord and Christ."

When the people heard this, we were cut to the heart and asked Peter and the other apostles, "Brothers, what shall we do?"

Peter replied, "Repent and be baptized, every one of you, in the name of Jesus Christ for the forgiveness of your sins. And you will receive the gift of the Holy Spirit. The promise is for you and your children and for all who are far off—for all whom the Lord our God will call."

I leaped towards Peter, shouting, "ME! Baptize me! I believe! At last I believe!" I went with the others, was baptized, and proclaimed my belief that Jesus is the Christ to all who would hear.

That's why I had to stop you, even though I don't even know who you are. Don't be a simpleton like me, denying the truth before my face. As for me, I had a miracle before my very eyes, and yet I could not see it for what it was. I thought Jesus healed my son so I would believe He was powerful or so the people in Caesarea Philippi would know God had sent a prophet. But it was so much more. It wasn't about healing my son's body; it was about healing all our spirits. God was about so much more than pleasing a father by healing his son. He was about elevating His Son to sit at His mighty right hand and pouring out His Holy Spirit on all who will receive Him.

Look around! Can you see it? Can you see the impact

the Holy Spirit has made, just today, on the lives of Jews in Jerusalem? This is just the beginning! You'll see! Don't wait! *Don't doubt!* **Believe!**

1. *When the doubting man said "if", Jesus and everyone present knew he had doubts. What do you think of Jesus' reaction to the father's doubts? What do you think Jesus' reaction is to your doubts?*

2. *All Christians have times when they doubt what Jesus can do, why He's doing something or even who He is. Has cancer given you doubts? If so, what are they?*

3. *Take a moment to write a prayer, placing your doubts at Jesus' feet.*

4. *"God did this so that men would seek Him and perhaps reach out for Him and find Him, though He is not far from each one of us."* (Acts 17:27)
   What does this verse mean to you?

The Dead Man

John 11:1-44; Isaiah 6:1-7

𝓔verywhere I go, people always stop and ask me, "Are you *the* Lazarus? The one who died?" It happens all the time! Whether I am buying figs in the market or rushing to synagogue, a stranger will suddenly ask me, "Were you really dead?"

I answer, "Yes, I was really dead." It's an outrageous claim, but it's entirely true. So you think I am a fool to tell them I'm *the* Lazarus? Why shouldn't I? After all I've seen, do you think King Herod's guards or the High Priest's spies scare me? No way! You must not understand what happened when I died. Sit with me. I will tell you things that your mind cannot comprehend.

It all began with Jesus; every great story does. Jesus and I were close friends. Many times Jesus visited my home, and my sisters welcomed Him as if He was a beloved member of our family. We loved Him, and He loved us. That's why everyone was so surprised when I became ill and Jesus did not come. I was bedridden and delirious, so I know little of this time, but my sisters Martha and Mary were beside themselves with worry. We all knew that Jesus could heal me if He came, but after they sent word, Jesus didn't come. My body grew continually weaker. Then one evening, I died. I was buried in the tomb on the hills beyond Bethany. Really! Just beyond that rise. They tell me it was a lovely service, but it pains me to think of the agony my sisters went through.

I can see it in your eyes—you want to ask me about what happened. Most people are too hesitant to ask, but I know you want to hear it all. Go ahead; ask me, "What was it like when you died?"

I have told this many times, so I know there are no words to explain it, but I will try. After I died, I was in the temple of the Lord, something like our temple in Jerusalem, and yet not like it at all. It was much the way the prophet Isaiah described hundreds of years ago. Everything was glowing with a light more radiant than white. The Lord God Almighty was sitting high on His throne, and the train of His robe had no end. It filled this magnificent temple as far as the eyes could see.

Then I heard the singing, so rich and full you could touch it. Music resonated from every direction, yet somehow I knew it was the seraphs' voices I was hearing. The spectacular six-winged angels rose behind the throne, singing, *"Holy, holy, holy is the Lord Almighty; the whole earth is full of His glory!"*

As the seraphs called to each other, the doorposts and

thresholds shook, and the temple was filled with smoke.

In an instant, I was overwhelmed by my own sinfulness. Everything in this place was pure and clean but me. There I stood, a mere sinful man in the presence of our perfect and all-powerful God. Washed with the despair of every unfit thought, word, and deed I had ever committed, I dropped to my knees and hid my face in the floor. "I am unclean!" I cried in bold-faced fear. "I cannot survive in Your holy presence! I must surely die."

But like Isaiah, an angel came and placed a coal from the Holy altar on my lips and said, "See, this has touched your lips; your guilt is taken away and your sin atoned for."

And with a breath, it happened. Every guilt, every shame, all my bitterness and anguish were gone. It was as though they never existed. All that was left was me, humble Lazarus, filled entirely with the glory of the Lord. The Lord's glory was no longer something surrounding me; it was all that I am. It was the whole of my being. Words of praise flew from my heart unceasingly. I could not have stopped my praising even if I wanted to, and that's when I heard it.

"What?" you ask. "What could have intruded on the Lord's throne room?"

It was Jesus' voice. His voice has always been a sound of joy to me. He speaks with such depth and warmth in all He does. But this time, His voice was like a screech on a soundless night. I was standing before the throne of

God, filled with His glory, and I heard from somewhere beyond the temple, Jesus saying, "Take away the stone."

Although I heard Jesus, I could not comprehend what was happening. My sister Mary's voice responded, "But, Lord, by this time there is a bad odor, for he has been dead four days." Were they speaking of *my* tomb and *my* body? It seemed impossible, because I stood there singing praises, filled with more joy than a human body could possess.

Then Jesus said, "Did I not tell you that if you believed, you would see the glory of God?"

Then from behind me, a small wave of darkness rolled toward where I stood. From the darkness I heard Jesus talk to the throne before me, "Father, I thank You that You have heard me. I knew that You always hear me, but I said this for the benefit of the people standing here, that they may believe that You sent me."

I turned toward Jesus' voice. This time I heard Jesus shout, "Lazarus, come out!" As I walked towards Jesus, I realized I was still wearing my burial shroud. My hands and feet were wrapped with strips of linen, and a cloth was still around my face. There were others with Jesus, and He said to them, "Take off the grave clothes and let him go." As they uncovered my face, I knew that I walked from a tomb and was greeted by my sisters and loved ones, crying as they embraced me.

I felt the glory of the Lord leaving my body, and a dark emptiness filled me as I longed to return to God's presence. But then I turned, and there was Jesus standing before me, shining with all the glory I had just seen sitting on the throne of God. The darkness inside me left as I felt Jesus' light. What I had already known was now completely visible to me: God had sent His glory and radiance here to earth in the body of His Son, Jesus Christ.

Today, I look at those around me and I know they don't understand. They think that Jesus raised me from the dead to show His power, but nothing could be further from the truth. Jesus didn't raise me from the dead to prove He's powerful enough to defeat Herod and Pilate's troops, then prance into Jerusalem and proclaim Himself king. This wasn't about power; it was about glory—God's glory. Here on earth—in His Son, Jesus the Christ.

Of course, not long after I was raised from the dead, Jesus was crucified. With all that I knew and all that I understood, I did not foresee this. Jesus dying on the cross left me with doubts. I knew Jesus could conquer death; He had done this for me. But would He do it now? Not everyone He met was healed and not every deceased loved one was raised from the dead. He certainly had the power to overcome Pilate and Herod and avoid the cross, but He didn't. Perhaps I understood better than anyone that without a victory for Jesus, we were doomed. Who will be our champion in heaven if Jesus is not victorious on earth? Who will stand with us before God's throne as we are engulfed in every black, ugly sin we have ever committed? Who is holy enough to approach the altar of

God and take a coal from its eternal flame? Who is pure enough to cleanse us?

I could not sleep after I heard of Jesus' death. Then, after the Sabbath, joyful news came: *JESUS WAS ALIVE!* Jesus, in all His glory, has conquered not only death, but also life! I died the simple death of a man. But Jesus was the perfect Son of God. He had the power to stop His death a thousand different ways, but He didn't. Since Adam and Eve, God has waited for His Chosen One to place Himself on the altar to pay for our sins. Only a perfect sacrifice could save mankind. Jesus had no sin; He laid down His life for all who have sinned. Jesus has conquered my sin so I can live my life in peace, not fear.

Each day for me is filled with great anticipation. I look forward to the day I will die and arrive in the throne room again. Only this time there will be no fear, because Jesus has made me pure and clean by His blood. Go, good friend. Live your life fearlessly. Live in great anticipation of your visit to the throne room of God. *HALLELUJAH!*

1. *What do you think it was like for Lazarus to leave the glory of God's throne room for earth? How would you feel if this happened to you?*

2. *Imagine standing in the throne room and suddenly becoming aware of your sinfulness before the perfect*

holiness of God. Now imagine Jesus making you clean and pure. Wonderful, isn't it? Jesus has already taken care of this for all believers when He died on the cross. Write a thank you note to Jesus for preparing you for the presence of God.

3. *Before He raised Lazarus from the dead, his sister Martha had doubts. Here is Jesus' response to her doubts and ours:*

"Jesus said to her, 'I am the resurrection and the life. He who believes in me will live, even though he dies; and whoever lives and believes in me will never die. Do you believe this?'"
(John 11:25-26)

What does this verse mean to you?